GW01451652

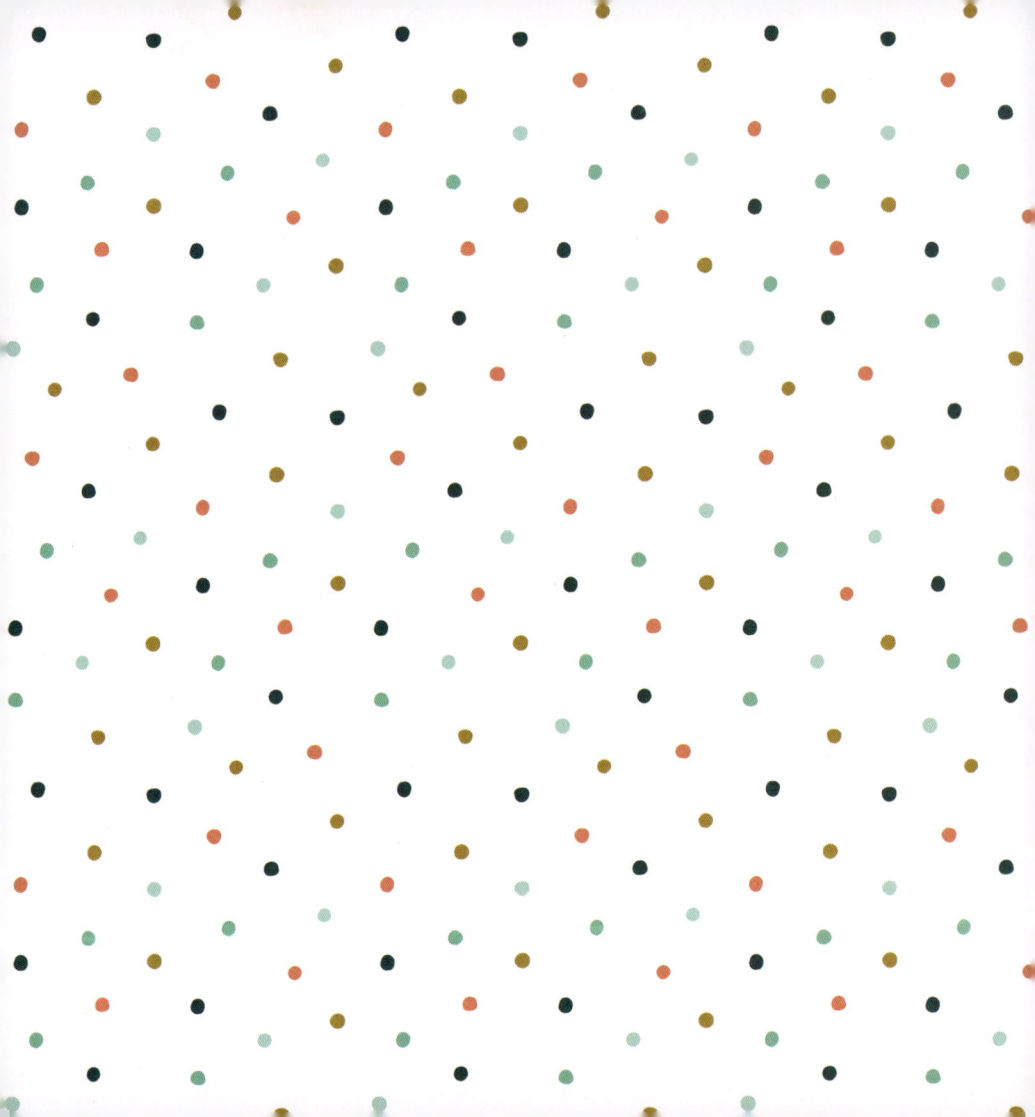

MUM TO MUM

PASS IT ON

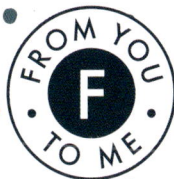

MUM TO MUM
PASS IT ON

Having a baby is a life-changing experience and you may feel a little overwhelmed and unsure. You are not alone.

Written by mothers just like you – for mothers just like you. This book is a precious gift full of practical tips and inspiration to help make your transition to motherhood smooth and stress-free.

The perfect gift to inspire and offer comfort to a new mother or mother-to-be.

BIRTH

Think of your birth plan as a set of birth preferences. It's okay to change your mind or even throw it away.

Register with all the baby-related websites and sign up for free gifts and discount vouchers.

Buy a toy comforter and take it
to bed with you for a few nights
before giving it to your baby. Your
smell is a great comfort to your
baby when he sleeps.

Write a list of things you will and won't do. For example, 'I won't use a dummy'. Review the list every three months or so and either laugh or get back on track!

Buy a pack of colourful muslin cloths or sew a little coloured ribbon onto plain ones. This will prevent them getting mixed up with other people's and reduce the risk of spreading germs from other children to your baby.

The baby's room can be finished after the birth. She will probably sleep in your room for at least the first six months, particularly if you're breast feeding.

Trust your instincts – if you're not happy, let someone know.

Hire, rather than buy, a TENS machine. They don't work for everyone.

Ask the midwife to place your newborn baby on your stomach after giving birth to allow skin-to-skin contact. Your baby will crawl up towards you – it's amazing.

Your legs might shake uncontrollably during labour. It's common, so don't panic.

If you have swollen ankles, they may take a few weeks to go down after the birth, but they will.

Take lots of photos and videos. Children grow up so quickly and you can never capture those precious images and moments again. Regularly back up the files from your computer and once a year try to make a photo book/album.

It's not unusual for babies to have all kinds of patches, marks, rashes and spots on their skin. Try not to worry, it usually sorts itself out.

The name you have chosen for your baby is perfect.

You may be a bit forgetful after you give birth, so when you're given a birth present, capture it on the back of the card. That way, you will remember who gave you what when it comes to writing thank you notes.

If you're given lots of newborn clothes as presents, take some of them back and exchange them for a bigger size. Your baby will grow so quickly in the first six months and he won't need them all.

Night sweats for a few weeks after giving birth are common. Tuck a muslin cloth under your pillow and use it to wipe yourself during the night.

FEEDING

Breastfeeding can take up to six weeks to really get the hang of. Try to stick it out, but if you can't, then don't worry.

If you're breastfeeding, make sure you eat regularly and well. You also need to drink lots of water, so leave bottles of it around the house and top them up each night before you go to bed.

Keep a stack of healthy snacks by
your bed and in your bag to top
up your energy levels during feeds
– dried apricots, raisins, almonds,
bananas and energy bars are ideal.

Savoy cabbage leaves really are fantastic for soothing sore, engorged breasts – provided you don't mind the smell. They're also the perfect shape.

To remember which breast you need to feed from next, buy a small elasticated bracelet. While you are feeding, move it to the other arm so you know which breast to use for the next feed.

You don't need to buy a breast pump. They can be hired. Check with your doctor or health visitor for schemes in your area. Always opt for an electrical one – they're much more efficient.

If your nipples are really too painful, express your milk for a couple of days and give yourself a chance to recover.

Try not to continually stare at your baby while you're feeding because it will give you a stiff neck and backache.

Wind your baby gently and if they haven't brought up the wind within ten minutes, then they aren't likely to. Put them down and if they seem uncomfortable, try again.

Help your baby learn to sleep through the night. When your baby wakes for night-time feeds, use a dim light and don't stimulate her by talking.

Clean any sick on carpets and furniture immediately as the baby's stomach acid will take the colour out of the fabric and cause a stain. Rub with cold water to remove the protein before washing as hot water cooks the protein, making it hard to remove.

Buy a plastic tub for measuring formula and prepare the milk powder for your feeds in advance – this saves time and effort, particularly if you have had a disturbed night.

You don't need to warm the milk for your baby. Give it to them cold or, if using cartons, at room temperature and they will get used to that. You then won't have to worry about finding a place to warm feeds when you're out and about.

Buy a cheap, second kettle for making up bottle feeds. You can boil the water and leave it to cool without someone accidently reboiling it and leaving the water too hot to make up the feed.

Once your baby starts crawling and putting things in their mouth you don't need to sterilise everything every day, just make sure they are thoroughly cleaned.

WEANING

Buy a simple highchair (you really don't need height adjustments, drink stands or the ability to tip the seat backwards) and make sure it fits up to the table for family mealtimes.

Make your own messy mat for under the highchair by buying a metre or so of plastic table covering. This can later be used to cover the table during toddler painting or messy play.

Babies wean at different rates so
be guided by your child rather
than comparing with your friends.
If your baby isn't ready, try again
in a week or two.

Try to eat at the same time as your child to encourage positive behaviour. Talk to them about the day's activities rather than food or eating and encourage good table manners.

Eat meals at the table and make
indoor picnics a special treat.

Discourage fussy eating – don't offer an alternative meal and don't give them any pudding if they refuse to eat their main course. Also, avoid filling them up with bread. They won't let themselves starve.

Cook more food than you need for one meal, and then make a second meal with the addition of beans or pasta.

Once weaning starts, encourage your baby to wash their hands before and after meals so that it becomes part of their routine.

If your child doesn't appear to like a certain food, wait a few weeks and try again. The chances are, they will eat it.

If your baby is refusing to eat, it might be because they're not hungry. Move the mealtime to half an hour later and try again.

Teach your child to use a straw as soon as possible – a valuable skill for giving drinks on the move and cartons of milk when you forget the bottle.

When you visit a store that provides disposable bibs, ask if you can take an extra one and pop it into your bag for emergencies.

At mealtimes or parties, put savoury food out first and only bring out the cakes and biscuits when all the children have finished eating their main meal.

Encourage a reluctant eater
by inviting a little friend
(who eats well) to tea.

Get your toddler involved in creating the meal so that they know what went into it and they will be pleased to eat what they have made.

Toddlers' taste buds change at around the age of two, so don't be surprised if they suddenly stop liking certain foods.

If your child won't drink milk, then offer them cheese, yoghurt, fromage frais, milky puddings, custard, tinned sardines, mashed salmon, ice cream, tofu, bread, muffins, baked beans, lentils or chickpeas as these contain high quantities of calcium.

If your child doesn't like fruits, disguise the fruit by puréeing it and adding it to custard, yoghurt or fromage frais.

Make fruity lollipops by juicing fresh oranges and freezing the juice in plastic lollipop moulds.

If your child doesn't like vegetables, disguise them by puréeing them and adding to a casserole or pasta sauce.

Keep a packet of freezable yoghurts in the freezer for lunch boxes. They help to keep the container cool and will have defrosted by lunchtime ready for eating.

CHANGING

Tell your baby what's happening to her. "I'm going to change your nappy/clean your teeth/give you some milk." No one likes to be grabbed and forced to do something, so let them know what's going on.

When you change your baby's nappy, put a clean nappy underneath the dirty nappy to catch any accidents during the change process – it's much easier than doing a full outfit change.

Distract a wriggly baby during nappy changes by giving them something safe to play with.

Make an effort to always change your child's nappy in your bathroom – that way they will grow up knowing that this is where they go to the toilet.

Use a large towel to make a cosy, washable cover for cold changing mats.

Give your child appropriate words to use to describe passing a motion. This will make toilet training easier as they will know the language to use.

There's no rush to toilet train. Wait until your child is ready and don't be driven by other people – it's not a competition.

If your child tells you they don't want to wear nappies anymore (particularly night-time nappies), seize the opportunity. Let your child take the lead on when they're ready for potty training.

There are likely to be accidents at night when toilet training – use a layering system of absorbent sheets and cotton sheets so that a layer can be removed if the bed is wet. A spare duvet is also a good idea.

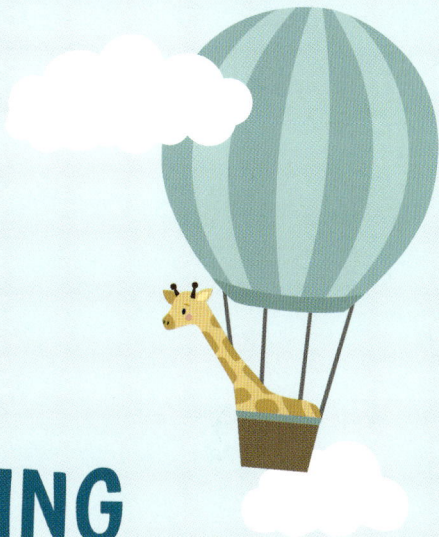

CLOTHING

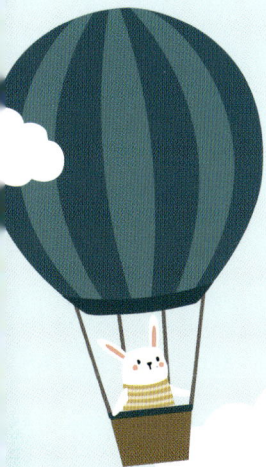

Buy the vests that have a cross over flap at the shoulders. These open wide enough so that the vests can be taken off/put on over the body, rather than over your baby's head. Particularly useful with an explosive nappy!

Socks have a habit of coming off small babies, so when it gets really cold, put tights on under trousers rather than socks.

Baby clothes with buttons or bows on the back can irritate a baby and prevent them from sleeping properly. Avoid buying them and exchange any that are given as gifts.

Buy packs of socks in the same colour or two packs of mixed colours – one always goes missing, so at least you will be able to make a pair and have a spare!

In the first two years, your child doesn't need more than eight outfits at a time. Children grow so quickly, they won't wear anything out.

6 to 9 month clothes are only millimetres smaller than 9 to 12 month clothes so, where you can get away with it, miss out the 6 to 9 month range and buy bigger. You will get better value for money.

If you're lucky enough to receive a present for your baby in a cloth drawstring bag, use this to keep a spare set of clothes together for your child when you go out.

Clothes can fit again once your toddler stops wearing nappies and loses baby chubbiness, so don't be too keen to get rid of their little outfits.

Sell grown-out-of, clean and good quality outfits, toys and bottles, as well as excess nappies. Try to sell the clothes according to the season to maximise the price.

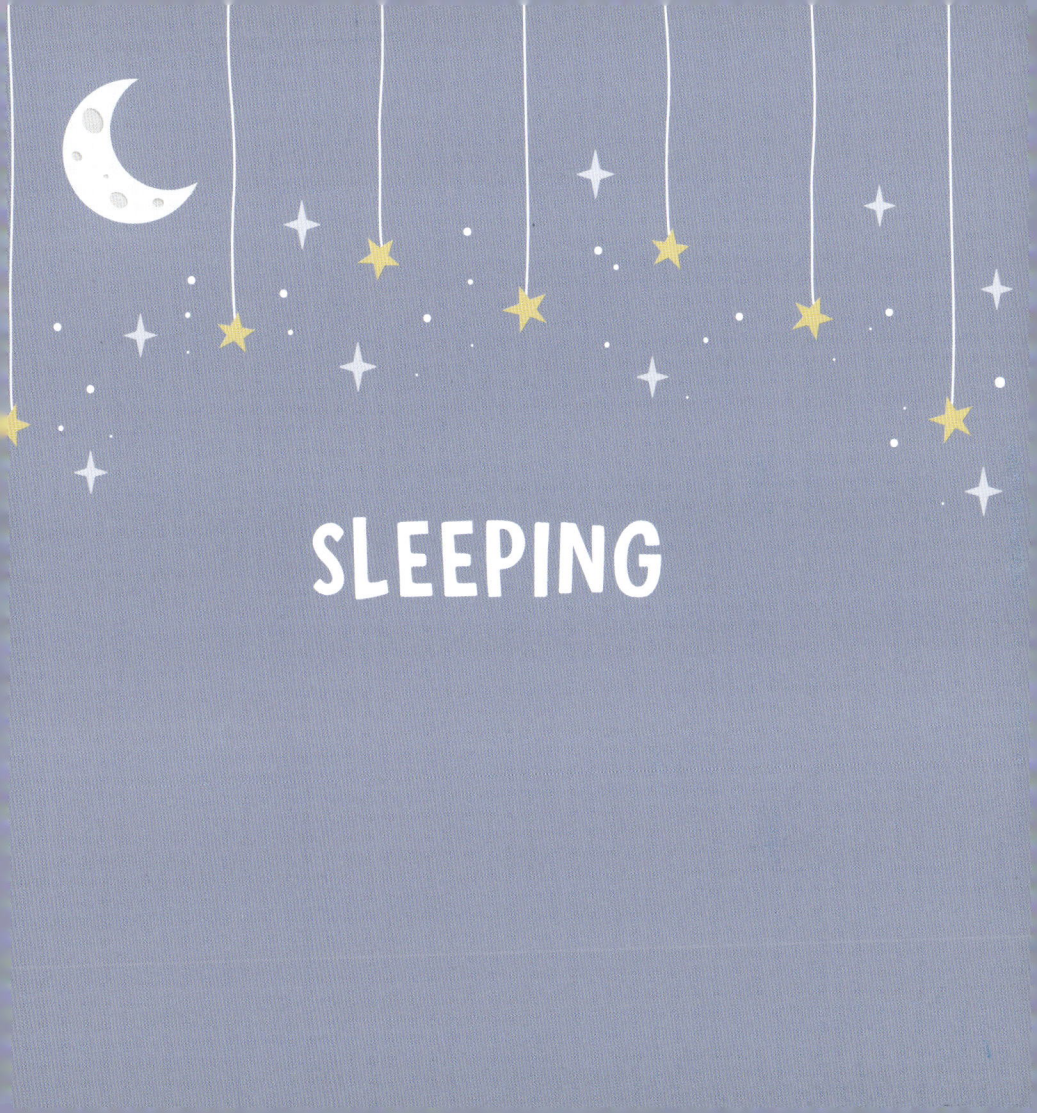

SLEEPING

Buy a basic baby monitor. You don't need a video screen, music, intercom or lights because you will never use them.

Buy three soft toy comforters: one for bedtime, one for the wash and one as a spare, in case this important 'friend' is ever mislaid.

Only let your child have a toy comforter when they're in their cot. They will sleep with the movement of the car or buggy, and a lost comforter may mean no sleep for you all night.

Babies can make a lot of noise at night, so get used to their snuffles, gulps and snorts, and only get out of bed when they're really ready for feeding or need attention.

Have some quiet time with your baby before bedtime and give them their last feed in their darkened bedroom. This will calm them and help them to go to sleep more easily.

Do a baby massage course and massage your baby between bath and bed. It helps relax baby and make them sleepy.

At night-time, change your baby's nappy halfway through the feed rather than at the end of the feed. This will prevent him from being woken up too much just before you put him back to sleep.

Make a distinction between daytime and night-time naps so that your baby learns that night-time is a long sleep. You could do this by using a grobag at night and a blanket during the day.

The more interaction you have
with your child during the
day, the less time they will need
from you at bedtime.

It's two stories and then bed - and stick to it! The minute you do an extra one, you will always have to do it.

Leave your child's room purposefully so that they know it's time to sleep.

Make sure bedtimes are relaxed and read in a soft and calm voice. If possible, make the last one a sleepy bedtime story.

If your child won't settle into a routine at night or starts to buck the routine, get someone else (Dad, Grandma etc) to put them to bed for a few nights.

Be prepared to veer from the routine when they're ill, but reinstate it again when they're feeling better.

Once your baby reaches 10 months, she should be sleeping through the night. If she wakes up for milk, give her cooled, boiled water and soon she won't bother to wake.

If your child wakes in the night, stay calm, be firm and stick to your routine.

Make a glow-in-the-dark
picture with your child, it
will help to encourage them
into bed at night.

Try not to let nap times rule your day – you don't have to stay in the house. It's okay for them to sleep in the car, pram or buggy.

Once your toddler is approximately 18 months old, cut out the morning naps – one in the afternoon is enough. They will sleep better at night.

PLAYING

Second-hand toys are great value. Plastic toys, in particular, can be easily cleaned. Buying and selling on websites or through local papers is easy and you can pick up some real bargains.

Books or toys from a charity shop can be a lovely and very inexpensive treat.

Babies and toddlers need to learn
to play by themselves, so you
don't have to entertain them all
day long.

Give your child as much fresh air as possible – they will sleep much better.

Create models using tin foil, old toilet roll holders and paint – a cheap but fun exercise.

Make your own play dough.
It's very cheap and easy to do,
with recipes available on the
internet.

Save old clothes, hats and handbags, and keep them in a box for dressing up.

Old wallets with out-of-date round-edged credit/loyalty cards make great play things for toddlers.

Put different letters or coloured dots onto the back of jigsaws so that they can easily be separated when your toddler mixes all the jigsaw pieces, from different sets, together.

Make your own flash cards by cutting pictures out of magazines and sticking them to pieces of old birthday or Christmas cards.

Swap toys with another child for a few weeks so that your child gets to play with something different without having to buy it.

Swim nappies that haven't been soiled can be washed, dried and reused a couple of times to save money.

Get down on the floor and play with your child as much as you can. Take it in turns to lead the play and go along with whatever he comes up with.

LEARNING

Sew squares of different fabric together to make a sensual toy to stimulate your child.

Help your child get used to being alone (even for you to go to the toilet in peace) by leaving the room for increasing amounts of time. It can be started by playing peek-a-boo.

Use positive, encouraging language, for example, 'Keep your plate on the table' rather than 'Don't throw your food on the floor' which focuses on the negative behaviour.

Let your child have their own feelings. For example, don't tell them what they like/don't like, allow them to find out and express it for themselves.

When your child cries, these are useful responses: 'Some things are worth crying about – this isn't one of them.' Or alternatively, 'Some things are worth crying about – this is one of them.' And always treat them with empathy and cuddles.

Regularly check out your actions and laugh if you have fallen for a toddler trick – then do something about it. Playing for time to stay up late is a usual one.

Restrict your child to a set time for television or using the computer. Encourage them to draw, read a book or play games as a family.

Leave nursery school with conviction when you drop your child off – say goodbye and don't linger as this may upset your child.

When your child falls over and is hurt, don't tell them that the floor was naughty and smack it, your child may think that it's okay to smack/hit and that floors can be naughty.

When you read to your child, point to the words so that they learn to read from left to right and get used to this for when they start reading.

Teach your toddler to stand
still when you call out 'STOP'.
Invaluable when you need them
to stop and stay where they are.

Teach your child to only jump
into the swimming pool on a
certain unusual command such as
'bananas' so that they don't just
jump into water.

Teach your child a special word to indicate that they need to come and find you. Invaluable when they decide to play hide-and-seek when you least expect it.

Try to find a neutral place to send your child if she has behaved badly – avoid her bedroom as this needs to be a safe place where she feels secure and can sleep soundly.

Your toddler will learn colours easily if you describe objects in general conversation. For example, 'Here's the blue bowl' or 'Would you like your green cup?'

Encourage your toddler to count
by playing counting games –
count steps, red cars on a journey,
sheep in the field etc.

Be mindful of what you say in front of your children, they pick things up very quickly and it may come back to haunt you.

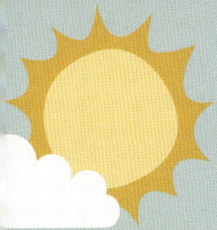
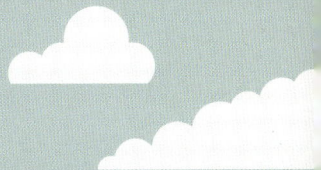

TRAVEL

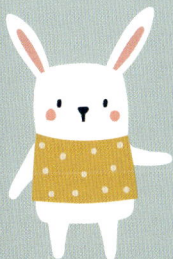
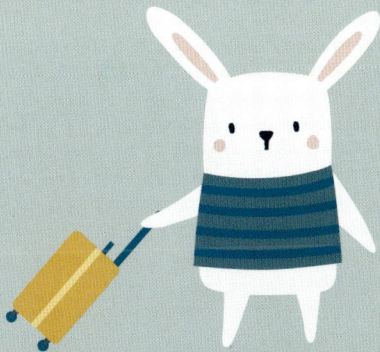

Research prams and travel systems for ease of use and weight. Make sure you can collapse, assemble and lift it easily and that it will fit comfortably onto buses and into your car. Try not to be swayed by design and gadgets.

Make a list of all the things you need to take with you for a day out – laminate it and attach it to your baby bag.

Allow lots of time for travelling, even if it's only to the shops. There will always be something unexpected, like a full outfit change or not being able to get the buggy up.

Keep a couple of nappies and a pack of baby wipes in the glove compartment of your car – you will forget your change bag one day.

Keep dried apricots, rice cakes and boxes of raisins in your car or bag for energy snacks during the day.

Put your child in the car
first and worry about the
shopping second.

Whenever you go away, buy a local postcard, date it and ask your child to draw or write on it. Then send it to yourself to keep a record of trips and how your child's writing changes.

Take a spare set of clothes for your child (and you if possible) on day trips. You will need them on at least one occasion!

Restaurants often give out small packs of pencils and colouring books – keep these in your bag for the times when you need your child to entertain themselves.

Take talcum powder to the beach.
Use it on sandy bodies to easily
remove the sand before putting
clothes and shoes back on.

Annual membership to a local attraction is usually a worthwhile investment. Children, particularly toddlers, don't mind if you go every week!

Read and record your child's favourite stories for your use only. They can play them over and over again at home.

Play dough is a good thing to take on long journeys such as train or plane trips. It's cheap and disposable, and keeps toddlers amused.

Put coloured ribbons on your bags when flying. To entertain your toddler, get them to help you spot the bags.

Try not to pack too much.
Children usually don't care if they
wear the same clothes again.
Split the clothes between bags
so that you all have something to
wear should a bag get lost.

YOU

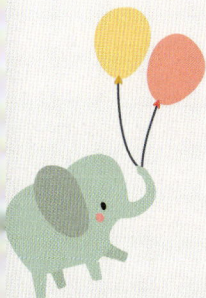

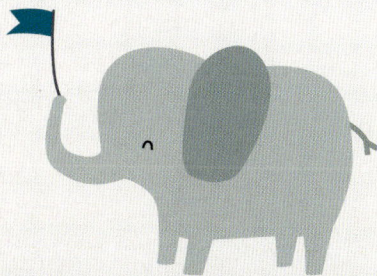

Invest in a moving musical mobile for your baby's cot – they usually play for up to 20 minutes which gives you enough time to have a shower, get dressed and feel human again.

Let your partner do some things their way with your child – you never know, you might learn something.

Go out with your baby as soon as you feel you can after giving birth. Your baby is really portable at this age and you really can do it on your own.

Accept invites for dinner and take your baby. The chances are, she will sleep through most of it anyway and you will get to enjoy some adult company.

Let yourself ask for help. It could
be the best thing you ever do.

Buy a calendar each year and use it to record key events for your child such as first tooth, sitting up, crawling etc. It's so easy to forget what happened and when.

Join a local postnatal group so that you meet other parents. They are going through the same things as you, and a problem shared is a problem halved.

Make a memory box for your child and fill it with mementoes, for example, first outfit, old favourite toys, newspaper clippings, etc. Explore the box with your child as they grow and ask them what they would like to add.

You can contact the doctor/ midwife/ health visitor as many times as you like. Call them if you're worried.

Buy several hand creams and put them all around the house. The constant handwashing makes your hands very dry and a good hand cream is a must.

It's alright to tell people to leave you alone to settle in when you have given birth. If they do come, ask them to bring a meal or something you need.

If you can (other children permitting), sleep when your baby sleeps – the washing-up can wait.

Trust your instincts. If you're worried about anything, get the appropriate help and a second opinion if necessary.

Your baby will learn to adapt to your lifestyle, so you don't have to be quiet when they are resting or having a sleep.

Grandparents can be a great help. However, it's okay to ignore their advice, particularly if you feel it's too much about the old days!

Capture all those precious
moments that are so easily
forgotten. There's an extensive
range of beautiful hand illustrated
memory journals at
www.fromyoutome.com

Join the local library and borrow books for you and your baby. For example, baby cookery books, relaxation books or just general reading.

Listening to nursery rhymes is great, but you can play your own music too. Your baby will enjoy being exposed to a variety of sounds and rhythms.

Once you have had the okay from the health visitor, get your figure back quickly by doing a set number of sit-ups or other exercises each time you change your baby's nappy. They love seeing you on their level and enjoy the movement.

If you can (other children permitting), sleep when your baby sleeps – the washing-up can wait.

Trust your instincts. If you're worried about anything, get the appropriate help and a second opinion if necessary.

Your baby will learn to adapt to your lifestyle, so you don't have to be quiet when they are resting or having a sleep.

Grandparents can be a great help.
However, it's okay to ignore their
advice, particularly if you feel it's
too much about the old days!

Capture all those precious moments that are so easily forgotten. There's an extensive range of beautiful hand illustrated memory journals at www.fromyoutome.com

Join the local library and borrow books for you and your baby. For example, baby cookery books, relaxation books or just general reading.

Listening to nursery rhymes is great, but you can play your own music too. Your baby will enjoy being exposed to a variety of sounds and rhythms.

Once you have had the okay from the health visitor, get your figure back quickly by doing a set number of sit-ups or other exercises each time you change your baby's nappy. They love seeing you on their level and enjoy the movement.

Keep a little jotter/notebook handy and write down all the funny things your child says – you easily forget.

Buy your nappies and baby products from shops that provide loyalty incentives and then spend the bonus points on nice things for you.

Stressed out by baby books and all the baby advice? Put them in a cupboard and trust your instincts. You can always get them out another day if you feel the urge.

Babysitters can be expensive,
so join, or set up, a babysitting
group with local mums.

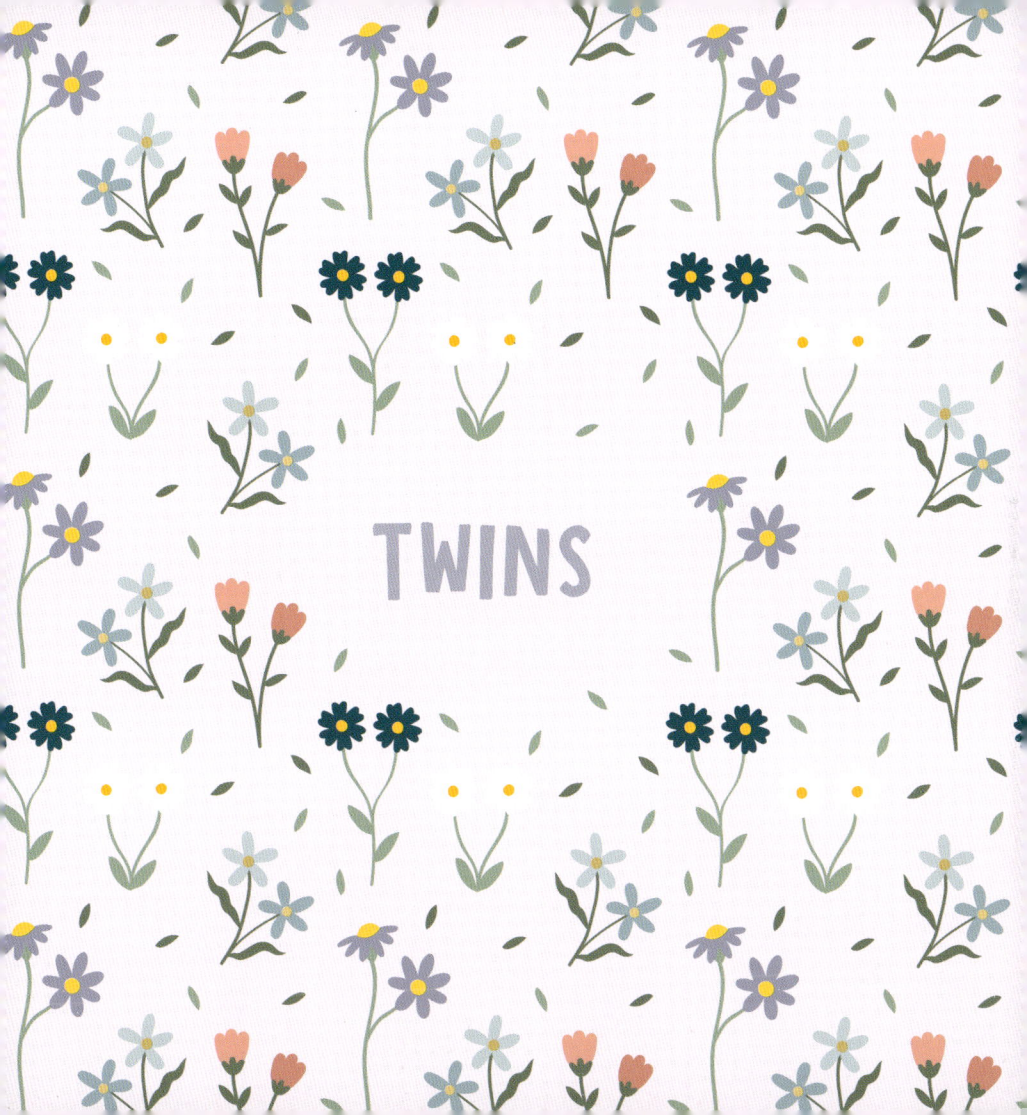

TWINS

Alternate bath nights for your babies. Put one in a bouncy chair to watch and spend quality time bathing just one baby.

Put your twins to sleep at the same time. They may wake each other up at times, but this will happen at any age, so the sooner they get used to each other's noise, the better.

To bottle feed twins at the same time, place them in bean bags as these hold the babies in a good position.

You don't need to buy two of everything when it comes to toys. Twins don't need any more toys than a single baby as they can only play with one thing at a time and it encourages sharing.

Join multiple-birth clubs and associations. These groups provide lots of great advice, support and information.

Accept all offers of help. If someone offers to take one baby for a walk – let them. It will give you one-to-one time with the other twin and helps her to learn to cope without the other.

My top tips to pass on . . .

Mum To Mum, Pass It On first published by **FROM YOU TO ME LTD,** in 2011.
This design published July 2023

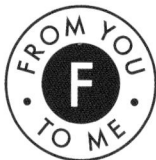

For a full range of all our titles where gifts can also be personalised, please visit

WWW.FROMYOUTOME.COM

FROM YOU TO ME are committed to a sustainable future for our business, our customers and our planet. This book is printed and bound at a contracted printer nearest the recipient, on FSC® certified paper.

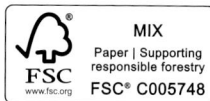

MIX
Paper | Supporting
responsible forestry
FSC
www.fsc.org
FSC® C005748

1 3 5 7 9 11 13 15 14 12 10 8 6 4 2

Copyright © 2011 & 2023 **FROM YOU TO ME LTD**

ISBN 978-1-907048-26-5

FROM YOU TO ME, STUDIO 100, THE OLD LEATHER FACTORY
GLOVE FACTORY STUDIOS, HOLT, WILTSHIRE, BA14 6RJ, UK

On a personal note

Helen Stephens became a first-time mother aged 41. Until then, she had undertaken a number of demanding and stressful jobs, but nothing had prepared her for the overwhelming, all consuming and exhausting role of a new mother.

Despite reading many books in preparation for the arrival of her daughter, Helen didn't find a single book that provided simple top tips that would make her life a little easier.

Based on her experiences, and with a little help from her friends, she has collected a wide range of practical tips and suggestions to save you from having to learn the hard way.

With a little help from her friends:

Vic, Cameron & Jamie
Sarah, George & Arthur
Debbie, William & Leo
Emily, Imogen & Benjamin
Faye & Billy
Sally, Poppy & Daisy
Marie, Arwen & Cainwen
Cathy, Oliver & Jack
Kerri, Eve & Jimmy
Julie, Xavier, Brodie & Asha
Charlotte, Sebastian, Gabriel & Cassius
Laura, Oscar & Isabelle

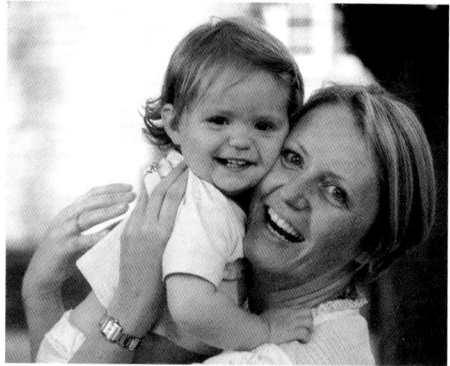

Míla & Helen

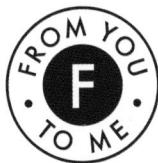